It's the Sugar, Stupid.

PATRICE ALEVY

It's the Sugar, Stupid.

ISBN: 1548770477
ISBN-13: 978-1548770471

CONTENTS

FOREWORD

This foreword will be short and sweet - the only sweet thing in this book.

With *It's the Sugar, Stupid*, I'm certainly *not* calling anyone stupid. "It's the sugar, Stupid," is my own personal daily mantra to myself.

By trying out some of the simple suggestions in this book, you could be experiencing the same life-changing results that I did in less time than it takes to figure out that the meds don't work!!

I'm not a doctor, a scientist, or health care professional. I'm just another person who was diagnosed with Type II diabetes. I was told to pop a couple of pills, shoot up some insulin and voila…normal blood sugar!

What I found was that nothing could be further from the truth - or our health.

I couldn't tolerate the meds I was prescribed (they made me violently ill). They did nothing to change my condition.

I had to find another way., and I did. After lowering my own blood sugar to healthy levels with no meds and no insulin... and losing 20 lbs. with no effort... in a short 3 months... my conclusion is that the mainstream medical community does *not* have it right! If they did, there would be no need for this information.

This book is about the easy and very accessible ways I got off the meds, controlled my numbers, and turned my health completely around in a very short amount of time.

Far from being stupid, reading this book may be one of the smartest decisions you ever make.

ACKNOWLEDGMENTS

I used to roll my eyes when I read acknowledgements…not anymore!

Writing a book about reversing diabetes was more difficult than doing it. Sometimes people have an idea and they don't know what to do next. That's what happened to me with this book. I knew I wanted to share my experience but really needed some expert advice. Then I shared the idea with my friend Rich DiGirolamo and he helped break it down into simple steps. Before I knew it, I was writing, rewriting, and being pushed to (sometimes uncomfortably), come up with cover designs, and all the stuff that goes into writing a book. He really didn't want any mention here. Ridiculous, people who were an integral part of something this important certainly need a mention. You should check him out at http://recessatwork. com. Thanks Rich!

Speaking of people who didn't want to be mentioned: Suzanne Lefcourt Harris. Suzanne edits and writes all kinds of copy for a living. She's busy, she has a family, and she recently went through a very trying time in her life. I mention this because SOMEHOW she found the time and the generosity of spirit to edit this book. I begged her not to because she really didn't need the extra burden. Her reply, "If I read the book and find a typo, it will kill me!" Thank goodness for her OCD with the written word, her friendship, her encouragement, and most of all, her original comment when I first told her about my healing journey: "You should start journaling what you're doing." The rest as they say... If you need an editor, you can contact her at https://suzanneharriscv.wordpress.com.

A huge thank you to Kristine and Doug Marsh. Doug for designing the cover, Kristine for generously volunteering his services.

I wouldn't have written this if not for my daughter Nikki. I also wouldn't have gotten gestational diabetes. Thanks kid!

My brother Jeff who supported me, encouraged me, and who calls me, "his brother in a sister's body."

Lastly, my husband Omar. Thank you for giving me the candy in the airport, you almost cashed in on the life insurance.

INTRODUCTION

If you are taking one or more medications for Type II diabetes, but you're not exactly thrilled with your results, you're not alone.

Medication for diabetes is now coming under fire the way Fen Phen, the popular weight loss drug, and Vioxx, the arthritis medication, both did. It's no wonder.

Millions of people across the country are experiencing many nasty side effects—and virtually no improvement in their health.

In fact, many people who have been on meds for years are actually in *worse* condition now than they were when they first heard the words "You've got Type II Diabetes" from their doctors.

What is going on??

Well, Type II Diabetes is a complicated, multi-faceted condition which requires a good hard look at our lifestyles.

The fact is, Type II Diabetes didn't even exist until the 20th century.[1] It wasn't until the 1980s that its rate started to rise alarmingly fast.[2]

Today, Type II diabetes is the seventh leading cause of death in the US.[3] What happened? Why is everyone getting diagnosed with this life-changing nightmare?

Ready to take the "die" out of diabetes?

If you are okay with staying on meds or insulin without making lifestyle adjustments, that's fine with me. I make no judgements—I'm no angel or

---

[1] American Diabetes Association http://www.diabetes.org/research-and-practice/student-resources/history-of-diabetes.html

[2] World Health Organization http://www.who.int/bulletin/volumes/89/2/11-040211/en/

[3] Medical News Today http://www.medicalnewstoday.com/articles/282929.php#diabetes_causes

genius myself. Let me assure you right now: You don't have to change anything you're doing.

All I'm asking you to do is read this book. Because you will probably pick up one tip that will make your journey easier. That's why I'm writing this. I'm not here to change you or to brainwash you into some radical mindset, diet, or lifestyle.

I've got dozens of little ways that I know can help. You might find just one thing that relieves diabetic nerve pain, lowers your numbers a bit, or just makes you feel better.

I've also included steps you can easily take right now. Remember: the debilitating effects of diabetes won't wait and neither should you.

Let's go.

Chapter 1

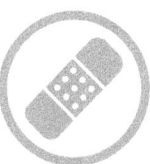

My Ridiculously Fast Healing Timeline

My numbers in June

I was diagnosed in June of 2016 with a fasting blood sugar of 324 and an A1C of 12.

Scary, right?

If you're reading this for someone else and are not familiar with these numbers, 324 is approximately 224 points too high.

The A1C is a marker that measures the glucose in your blood by assessing the amount of something called "glycated hemoglobin."

The medical community would like your numbers to be below 5.7. That should give you a good indication of how high mine was.

What happened in August

Two months after my diagnosis, in August, I noticed that a wound on my shin had suddenly healed. I'd had that wound for many, many months.

What had changed? I felt like a huge moron for not making the connection between a wound that wouldn't heal and diabetes, but it was completely healed.

A few weeks after that, I noticed that the heels of my feet once again looked like they belonged on a human and not a reptile.

What happened in September

One month later, I went back for a blood test in September. My A1C had dropped to 6 and my cholesterol went from 293 to 170.

...and in October

Another month later, in October, I went to the dentist. The hygienist was astonished at the improvement in my teeth and gums.

WTF Happened?

I'm no math genius. And I'm not a health nut, a strict dieter, an exercise freak. Not a radical do this or that person either.

But in less than 6 months my body began dramatically healing. My mood, sleep habits, motivation, and mental clarity all dramatically improved too. No, it didn't happen without some action on my part. (That action is exactly what's in this book.)

But it was a lot easier and faster than any doctor, PA, book or website ever said it would be.

After years of having diabetes, *I turned it all around in six months*. That's a blink of an eye to see and feel such dramatic improvements.

If I can do it, so can you. And it's just one easy step at a time.

Don't get discouraged. Don't quit. Don't look back. Go.

Chapter 2

I Wept

"You have full blown diabetes, and you've had it *for years*."

I cried. I wept, actually because I was about to leave the country for two weeks. My family and I had been planning a trip to a tiny island in Colombia for a long time. This excursion was going to involve a few stops along the way.

Diabetes did *not* fit into my plans.

Yet there it was. My Physician's Assistant called me exactly *one hour* before we were leaving for the airport. UGH.

Apparently, my condition (Type 2) was long-standing and advanced. I had been experiencing symptoms (like leg pain and frequent tiredness) for years - without ever realizing what they meant!

The funny thing was that I actually already knew something about diabetes. I'd had gestational diabetes during pregnancy 18 years earlier.

But this was different. Full blown different.

I don't even know what the PA said. Something about giving me two different medications, something about side effects like nausea, diarrhea, gastritis, taking my blood sugar readings, eating, not eating... all the while listening with my hand over my mouth to stifle the sobs.

As soon as I hung up, my husband ran to the pharmacy to load up on all the meds I'd need for the trip.

I sat on the couch, too stunned to move.

Shoulda. Woulda. Coulda.

I began "should"-ing all over myself. I should have gone to the doctor sooner. I should've seen a symptom.

I should've not eaten this, should've eaten more of that, should've exercised more, less, added, taken away,

Stupid, stupid, stupid.

I should've known this would come back like the doctors told me it would, 18 years ago.

Betrayed. That's how I felt. Not betrayed by doctors or the medical community. I felt betrayed by my own body.

I now know that my body was doing what it's supposed to do, leaving clues and trying to find homeostasis—a fancy word for balance. *That's what all of our bodies do.* They try to tell us that we would benefit from doing some things—or a lot of things—differently.

Back to reality

But along with my husband, daughter, and her best friend, I had a plane to catch. I wanted to scream at them to let me stay home and be alone with my devastation. But I didn't.

I usually love airports. Not this time. Aside from my emotional state, I suddenly viewed everything I used to eat and drink as the enemy... the last bite or sip that would send me into a diabetic coma.

Dramatic, I know. But I was a hot mess.

I had the presence of mind to buy some hard candy. Even through my panic, I recalled the PA telling me to keep some with me in case my sugar dropped too low at some point.

That turned out to be a decision that kept me from a 911 call in the Panama airport.

"No side effects"

As it happened, the people we were staying with in Panama are both doctors. I felt a bit safer knowing they would know how to advise me.

Even better, as it turned out, one of them was also taking one of the meds I was prescribed. She reported no side effects, which encouraged me as I was about to take my first pill that evening.

Um, well, not so much. Thank goodness there were two bathrooms in their house.

I'll skip the gross parts, but I will tell you that I felt like a grenade had gone off in my belly. The pain radiated to my back, legs, neck... anywhere a gas bubble can travel.

Breakfast of Champions

The next morning an extremely unhappy me dragged myself to the breakfast table. I HAD to eat (or so I thought). I would have preferred to have been dragged behind the car, that's how sick I already felt from the meds.

After breakfast, my family and I were back at the Panama airport to catch our flight to San Andres, Colombia. Most of the airport in Panama has been renovated very nicely… except, of course, for the ladies' room.

I was feeling very sick and really needed to find a bathroom. I somehow made it to the ladies' room, only to find 2 stalls—and a line out the door. I stumbled back to my seat at the gate and silently prayed that my embarrassing public disaster would only be to throw up (and not the other thing).

For that they would've had to call a HAZMAT team.

I suddenly remembered that my husband, who is an "amateur expert" in acupressure had shown me some points on my body to alleviate high blood sugar and other symptoms. Bad idea, really, really, bad idea.

As I applied pressure to the point associated with the pancreas, I began to sweat and shake. I threw myself on the floor because I knew I was about to pass out anyway.

This must be a somewhat frequent occurrence in that airport as no one even looked up. After several candies that my husband retrieved from my purse, and 3 more attempts at floor gymnastics, I was able to board the plane and use the bathroom.

Didn't do the acupressure thing again until I got home.

Worse than cancer

The next two weeks were not fun healthwise, but I did manage to stay off public floors.

One of my husband's relatives who we were visiting in Colombia is a nurse. She told me that many doctors consider diabetes to be a worse fate than cancer because you can never be rid of it.

This is a theory that I am obsessed with disproving. As it happens, I am well on the way to doing just that, and so have many others.

We flew from the "big" island (13 miles around) to the smaller island (4.35 miles around) of Providence. We were going to be there for nine days. Need I say more?

When I saw the shospital (not a typo - it was a combination of shack and hospital), I suddenly became *all* religions. I didn't care who or what I prayed to, I just had to *not* have an emergency so I could stay out of that shanty built in 1920.

I made it home a few pounds lighter. No harm in that—except I would have preferred to lose weight some other way.

That's when the real fun began.

Glucometers,

strips,

lancets,

sore fingers,

multiple doctor visits,

changing and adjusting meds...

and lying to my doctor about taking my statins for high cholesterol.

I'll tell you why I lied to my doctor in a bit. I am also putting all my methods and suggestions for you in one place at the end so you won't have to highlight, mark pages, or go back and search for something that you feel might help you. You're welcome.

If you are reading this for yourself or someone else then you already know that our bodies are interconnected systems, much like the canals in Venice. Often when something is out of whack, it effects other things like blood pressure and cholesterol, or even thyroid.

And so I began the treacherous journey of researching cause and effect, reversing, and even healing diabetes. The amount of information is staggering. I watched PBS specials on blood sugar, I researched dozens of books, looked at numerous websites, all promising they had the one and only "cure."

Confused. Disheartened. Scared.

I read mountains of reviews on all the programs and books. In the end, I purchased nothing. Some of the information actually contradicted itself halfway through my reading. I was confused, disheartened, and not a little bit scared.

Go vegetarian,

vegan,

eat only organic,

no dairy,

lots of dairy,

exercise until you can't breathe,

don't overdo exercising,

meditate,

get rid of all stress (HA!).

Get rid of family members or friends that stress you out (double HAHA!).

Sleep at least 7 hours if not more every night, eat meat, no don't eat meat because it raises LDL levels, whey protein is perfect food but only if it is a certain kind, made with only solar cow's milk that is grass fed on an organic farm on a remote island in the South Pacific.

You get the idea.

The bottom line?

You are about to get your detective's license because you must be your own private diabetes detective. No one thing works for everyone across the board.

I am on a journey. A lifelong journey to optimize my years on this earth and feel as good as possible while I'm here. I'm also not going to bog you down with research findings, statistics, reports, etc… You can do that for yourself.

I want this to be as simple as possible to read and implement if you so choose. I won't be including "22 easy ways to bring blood sugar down," "11 secrets only doctors know about blood sugar," or "The best this" or "the worst that for diabetes."

Type II Diabetes is no joke and information should be clear, concise, and easy to read. That is my intention for myself and for anyone reading this.

First things first.

Let's discuss the most important organ in our bodies in relation to diabetes or any other unwanted bodily condition:

Our minds.

No, this is not a call to sit in a cave and meditate your diabetes away. Nor am I suggesting you need psychological help. Maybe you do. I don't know.

When this happened to me, I had to come to terms with the fact that I am the ultimate authority and decision maker when it comes to my health.

It also means the responsibility for my health rests solely on my shoulders, or pancreas in my case. This is really good news in my opinion. The doctors and nutritionists should be partnering with and supporting you. They cannot get inside my head or your pancreas to cure us.

But I can. And so can you!

So where do we start?

Well, for me it started with beating myself up. Don't start there.

So stop blaming yourself.

Stop with the woulda's and the shoulda's. It's a waste of your time and your energy.

You've got stuff to learn and stuff to do. Throw in being overweight, sedentary, and an unhealthy eater, and you really do need to get going now. Your journey to good health might take some time. The alternative might be….well you know.

What's your call to action?

Time is going to pass either way. I want my time here to be about feeling great and quality of life. This is a decision only I can make for myself and act on.

It was fine to have a good cry, and even indulge in some self-pity. Why me? But I knew I couldn't dwell there for too long because diabetes is a call to action.

I realized very quickly that a better question was "what" as in what am I willing to do to help myself? Cry while walking on a treadmill eating a celery stick??

(Obviously you don't want to eat while you're exercising because I don't want to get sued in case a stringy piece gets lodged in your throat.)

By the way celery is a great anti-inflammatory veggie. If you don't like it plain you can eat a piece of cheese with it, or nut butter with no added sugar for a great snack.

Easy steps you can take right now

Make up your mind that you will be *good to yourself* by following some or all of the suggestions in this book for a long, healthy life.

Take one small step at a time.

Most of all, *give yourself a high five* because you are already on your way just by reading this book!

Chapter 3

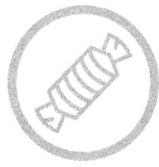

Craving Sugar

Years ago, I met an elderly gentlemen while waiting for my car to be serviced. I don't remember how the conversation got around to diabetes but he told me he healed his body completely eating ONLY fish and broccoli.

Do you see anything missing from that story?

SUGAR!

My sincere hope and intention for you is that you find a way to go one week without added sugar and very few carbs and see how your body stops craving those things.

I really want to be very clear about how much I craved sugar. I never believed that I could or would ever *not* crave sweets or carbs.

The true miracle for me? When I made the decision to get on the road to health *and stopped eating sugar, sugar* stopped eating at me.

I believe the same will be true for you. I've done too much research and heard from too many people to believe otherwise.

Ask yourself this: Is your life worth trying something for one week? If your answer is yes, then find a way to go *one week* without sugar.

This means no candy, cake, pastries, cereal, bread, pasta, rice, potatoes, fruit, etc... for one week. None.

Yeah, I know, a lot of diabetes resources are telling you that these foods are "OK" for you. But I'm telling you that the way I kicked diabetes really worked for me - and it worked *fast* and without drugs.

Believe me. If I can skip sugar and flour and carbs, you can do it.

For one week, just set your brain to accept that sugar *is not a choice and not an option.*

Be patient with the process and give it a chance.

As of this writing, it has only been 8 weeks since I have changed my eating habits.

My cravings, however, went away after only a few days.

Completely..

Again, I cannot emphasize enough that there is no single diet or exercise routine that will work for everyone. However, if you're patient—and can stay the course—you can stop the cravings.

I wish I could tell you that it will be easy or immediate but I would be extremely misleading, and even dishonest. Your individual process is also contingent upon how long you have had diabetes and the severity of your condition.

The effort is well worth it.

My husband brings home an occasional black and white cookie (my favorite). I now make him hide them so I'm not tempted.

You can do this too.

Your life may depend on it.

Easy steps you can take right now

Purge the pantry and fridge of all temptations so that you will have to get up and leave the house at midnight to get sugar/snack foods if a craving hits. Having kids is not an excuse to keep sweets around. They might not love it at first, but they will also benefit from less or no sugar.

I completely *disregard the diabetic guidelines because the foods listed there have way too many carbs and hidden sugars!*

Chapter 4

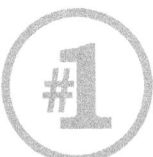

You Must Come First In Your Life

I have a friend with a history similar to mine. When she was pregnant, she had gestational diabetes. It returned as Type II many years later.

In spite of several different medications, her numbers were increasing and she wasn't feeling well. I had a rather strong discussion with her concerning her need to make her health her number one priority.

I will tell you the same thing.

I don't give a crap about laundry, cleaning, cooking, chores, errands, or anything else.

You must come first.

If you want to be able to take care of everyone else… you better take care of *you* first.

Poker... Family... STFU.

This same friend is one of those women who continually puts her family's needs before her own. I call BS on that, especially if your kids are older and self-sufficient. Many women can't seem to find the time to exercise... but will spend hours doing things for others.

Stop it!!!

My friend and I discussed how she couldn't resist the goodies being served at her poker games. I told her she either needed to stop going, find a way to not eat the junk, or host the game and provide the food.

As soon as she altered her eating habits, her numbers decreased significantly.

She still doesn't exercise regularly. But even without exercising - just making dietary changes - she is doing much better.

I still get in her face about her choices but I don't care. I want her in my life for a long, long time. I don't give a crap if that's selfish and you can consider yourself "told off" if you are taking care of everyone to the detriment of your own health.

Easy steps you can take right now

Tell your family you would love their cooperation and participation; however, you are going to take better care of yourself with or without their help or consent.

Jot down 3 things you are going to do to make your health a priority.

Some ideas: Rest when you're tired, shop for and make healthier food choices, and choose an exercise you can stomach and will do.

You'll have less stomach the more you exercise!

Chapter 5

Guidelines For Living

Once I decided to make peace with all this, I decided to follow a few guidelines for daily living. A balanced life encompasses several aspects. Healthy eating and exercise are only part of the equation.

As I mentioned previously, it's probably a stretch to get rid of everyone or everything that it is a source for stress in your life.

Believe me I understand that sometimes rolling out of bed is hard enough.

For me, I came to the realization that my *perception* of people or events was what produced stress, anxiety, or any other unwanted emotion. It's just like two eye witnesses giving two completely different descriptions of the suspect.

To paraphrase Shakespeare, only our thinking makes something "good or bad." In other words, *things have to change inside in order to change on the outside.*

Before I get started, I want you to know that I embarked on this journey without discussing it with the physician's assistant.

I just did it.

I have found that the medical community is not extremely receptive or supportive of anything not involving medicine or profits.

I have also read from many doctors that they are *not* taught anything about nutrition or dietary changes a patient must make if they are diabetic.

In addition, most have no clue regarding the latest cutting edge information concerning eating and exercising.

Having said that, you will find after each section that I advise you to check with your health care professional.

(Not because I think you have to. I just don't want to get sued.)

Meditation

These days there are many tools at our disposal to help us get a handle on stress. Many are completely free.

If you want to try your hand at relaxation/meditation you can google "15 minute meditations." So many will come up that you could do a different one every day for the rest of your life.

I like Dr. Deepak Chopra because he gives you a mantra to repeat which helps me quiet the mind chatter.

I also love to listen to Tibetan bowl meditations with rain or forest noises. I even put that on when I'm working on the computer or around the house. I have it on right now! I also love Native American flute music with rain/forest sounds.

I haven't levitated yet or experienced astro travel (haha) but I usually feel peaceful after listening. I prefer 10 or 15 minutes maximum. You might do 5 or 30, up to you.

I suggest if you choose to meditate, that you resist the urge to judge yourself or feel inadequate if the mind doesn't shut off. I don't even know if that's possible. I do know that the benefits are there whether they are immediately apparent or not.

Feeling peaceful even for a few moments can have long term effects on anxiety which in turn can positively impact your actions, emotions, and even sugar.

Easy steps you can take right now

Do a google search and see if any YouTube videos look interesting to you.

Look at your local library resources for free meditations classes.

Take a nice bath with bubbles and candles. Put on some soothing music and a do not disturb on the door. (Don't roll your eyes at me. I was also the multi-tasking, helicopter, control freak superwoman. If I could do it, you can do it.)

Now I don't give a crap if there's enough dog hair on the floor to make a cat. I've got that—and I also have a healthy body now.

Is it really that hard for you to choose happiness and health for yourself, as you do for everyone else in your life? Do it. It's your right to take care of yourself. You're the only one who can.

Chapter 6

Sleep

This is a complicated subject for most people. The official guidelines tell us that people who have diabetes must get 8 or 9 hours of sleep. I think that this is a very individual biological function.

Having said that, I can tell you that you shouldn't let yourself become exhausted or sleep-deprived because lack of adequate sleep places a lot of stress on your body. I find myself taking several days to recover from a night of no sleep.

Whether you sleep 6 hours or 10 is up to you. And guess what??

You don't have to check with the doc for this one!!

Easy steps you can take right now

Um…read the chapter title. I would opt for a bed or sofa but to each his own.

Seriously though, close the door and lie down for a nap. Ask for help and if no one is available to help with small kids, get in bed when they do and leave the unimportant stuff for another day.

Emotional Freedom Technique (EFT)

There is a technique called Emotional Freedom Technique (EFT), otherwise known as tapping. It has its roots in the ancient practice of acupuncture (without the puncture part).

In short, it is a technique that clears away your unwanted emotions because stuffing them down never works.

EFT brings them up, and clears them away with tapping on different parts of your face and body while repeating specific phrases. After the negative is voiced, positive statements are replaced to anchor them in your nervous system.

Google EFT for an in depth explanation and then go to Youtube to choose videos that resonate with you.

I like Brad Yates, GP Walsh, Margaret Lynch (mostly for finances), Carol Look, and Patricia Carrington. Again, see what, if any resonates with you. This is also totally free unless you choose to purchase a specific program.

Many of them like Brad Yates even have tap apps that you can download for one dollar. I always gravitate towards free or inexpensive, and anything I can do that doesn't involve a prescription.

I actually became a Level I practitioner after some fantastic results with tapping.

You can also find a local practitioner, do it over the phone, or via Skype if no one is local to you. I know a highly skilled tapping expert named Helen McConnell (*www.purposeprosperityhappiness.com*).

She is coming out with a new YouTube video called, "Tapping to Change old thinking."

Check out her site. You have nothing to lose but the unwanted cravings and emotional stuff.

Easy steps you can take right now

Get out your device and google EFT.

Read a few things and opt into a few, like Brad Yates. He gives tons of freebies.

Familiarize yourself with the tapping points on your body. Then tap, tap, tap.

I promise you, this is not voodoo. Many highly respected scientists and doctors attest to the efficacy of EFT/tapping Dr. Oz even did a segment on one of his shows.

Chapter 7

Get Out!

An excellent stress buster is to get outside with nature. Walk the dog, go by any body of water and take a walk, sit on your patio or balcony, whatever gets you outside every day for a while.

Sunlight infuses your body with vitamin D which many of us are deficient in. A few minutes is all you need to recharge.

I highly recommend escaping from the family for time on your own. Regardless of whether or not you choose to engage in some sort of exercise, get outside anyway.

I realize weather may play a part if it is a freezing winter or sweltering summer. However, going outside if you can is a great way to clear your head. If you absolutely cannot go outside, sit by the window and watch the beautiful snow, rain, or listen to the birds chirping.

By all means add to the list in whatever way works for you that doesn't include Snickers bars.

Whenever I'm feeling down, tired, or just out of sorts, I'm always happy I have to get the dogs out because I know I will feel better.

I always *do* feel better and the dogs are happy too. No fat dogs in my house!

Easy steps you can take right now

Any of the above suggestions would be appropriate right now. Obviously, if it's late at night, please take responsibility for your own safety.

If you rescue a large dog, feel free to get outside at night. They're better than an alarm. (The UPS people throw my packages from across the street when they hear my dogs!)

Chapter 8

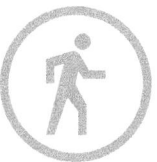

Exercise!

What's the best exercise for you? The one you'll do *consistently*?

This ties in with the previous segment very nicely.

A few ideas:

Rescue a dog from a shelter to walk and love,

treadmill,

exercise bike,

swimming,

yoga (not aerobic but still good),

roller blading,

elliptical,

join a gym and go to classes, and

my favorite… google, "walking at home."

There are many free exercise videos that involve nothing more than you and a little space in any room in the privacy of your home.

I love Leslie Sansone because she is always upbeat and has a variety of 1, 2, 3 or more equivalent miles of walking at home. There are others of course and I encourage you to find the ones you like best and do them at least 5 times per week.

It's free, it's convenient, and requires only a PC and you. That's it. I do some light weight lifting as well, because increased muscle burns fat and looks good on you.

A lot of local community centers offer a variety of free exercise classes as well. I love the dog idea because, well…I am a crazy dog person.

This next recommendation is a bit off the topic, but it's worth a mention. If you sit at a computer for many hours a day, consider getting a "standing desk." This allows you to stand at your work station, alleviating pain associated with sitting for extended periods of time. It's also been shown to increase productivity and posture. It is also recommended that you should get up every half hour and move around for 3 minutes to improve circulation and metabolism.

You can get an inexpensive standing desk on Amazon. To read more about this go to Dr. Joseph Mercola's website. He is a well-trusted authority on all subjects regarding health, exercise and nutrition. He also has wonderful products on his site but you don't have to buy any of them to get great info..

Obviously, you can add to this list. What you *can't* do is not do anything.

A moderate amount of exercise is so crucial and necessary that unless you are truly unable, you *must* find a way to exercise, whatever your favorite method. There's no getting around, under, or behind it.

If you want to control or reverse diabetes, there's simply no substitute for movement.

It is also the greatest stress buster there is. I recommend you mix it up a bit so you don't get bored and your body doesn't get too used to the same thing.

No, you cannot rely on medical professionals to inform you of the absolute necessity to exercise. But check with your doctor to confirm that you are fit enough to begin or continue an exercise program.

I feel this is worth repeating until you get it. *Some form of physical exercise is not optional!*

There are so many benefits to moving your body that I feel it is an obligation to make you understand that you must do something.

The latest information on exercising if you have diabetes is to take a walk for 10 minutes *after* every meal. This has been shown to be the most important time to move as it decreases your blood sugar readings by as much as 36%!!

Easy steps you can take right now

Find Leslie Sansone on YouTube, get up off your butt and do a one mile walk with her. It's fun!

Think of 2 or more ways you can exercise that will keep you interested and motivated.

You know what kept *me* motivated? My numbers kept decreasing and I lost 20 pounds with just a few changes.

Chapter 9

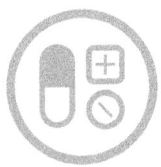

Supplements

This is another incredibly important subject—and one that will also require equal amounts of patience and caution.

I was so sick on the meds and not seeing the desired results in readings that I literally had no choice but to find alternatives.

I want to be absolutely clear about taking supplements while taking prescription meds, it is your responsibility to make sure you do your homework and check with your health care provider.

Some of the supplements I take have been clinically proven to lower blood sugar so effectively (with eating and exercise modification) that if you're not diligent you can get into real trouble as far as lowering your blood sugar too much while also taking medication.

Again, caution, due diligence, and very careful monitoring along with medical advice cannot be overstated.

Having gone on a rant about that, I never told my PA (I never actually saw an MD) what I was doing as I transitioned from Metformin, Onglyza, and

Glipizide.

My research and my own adverse reactions to these meds convinced me that I was on the right path for me. I slowly incorporated the supplements I am going to introduce to you.

Also, many health professionals are not informed as to the efficacy of using supplements.

Don't even get me started on Big Pharma, or the environmental impact of many meds. (Two thirds of the world's medicines come from rainforests, and that's another hot topic for me.)

Cinnamon

That's right. Cinnamon.

Not to be confused with cinnamon buns, rolls, cakes, or any other baked goods that includes a little cinnamon. (Don't shove a bun down your throat and then say I told you it was good for you!)

There are numerous studies on cinnamon that show a lowering of blood sugar throughout the day with just a teaspoon in the morning.

However, not all cinnamon is created equal. Ceylon cinnamon is the one that I take and I take it in the form of two capsules every morning.

I find this to be the most efficient and easiest way. You can also put it in tea, coffee, yogurt, or any other way you find palatable.

You can imagine how many results you will find if you google cinnamon. I'm going to tell you right now that I take 5 different supplements, and all of them come from Andrew Lessman's company.

Andrew Lessman has been making supplements for almost thirty years and has been on HSN for decades. I completely trust that his products are high quality and trustworthy. Andrew keeps up with the latest research and is always adding to his product line.

In addition, his plant uses only solar power to produce his vitamins. I love that he is environmentally conscious.

Of course, you are free to do your own research for any other company, however, I find it extremely convenient and comforting to know that he does all the science stuff while I just click and order.

When he has a presentation on the Home Shopping Network (HSN) shipping is almost always free. That's where I buy my cinnamon and the other products to follow.

A disclaimer: I am not affiliated nor do I get compensated for recommending these products. What I do get is healthy. Please check with your doctor.

Easy steps you can take right now

Look at *www.procapslabs.com*. You can also find his products on Amazon.

Order the cinnamon, or go to the health food store for Ceylon cinnamon, and incorporate a teaspoon a day in coffee, tea, or any other way you find palatable. It tastes nice sprinkled in coffee some heavy cream.

Turmeric / Curcumin

What? Never heard of them?

Get yourself to an Indian restaurant immediately!

These are spices that are used extensively in some cultural dishes in Asia. They are fabulous anti-inflammatory agents and are also wonderful for blood sugar.

There is a school of thought that all diseases stem from inflammation in our cells.

All of the supplements I use are multi-purpose for inflammation, blood sugar, blood pressure, and cholesterol.

As a great side benefit you may experience arthritic and diabetic neuropathy subsiding. Turmeric coupled with ginger is highly recommended for arthritis and joint pain. I take the amount recommended on the Andrew Lessman version's packaging which is one or more capsules daily with food.

Read the instructions when taking this or any supplement. Keep in mind that supplements might take a bit longer to work than synthetic meds. But the benefits are enormous. I personally eliminated all of the horrible side effects that I'd experienced from prescribed pharmaceutical medications.

If you cook with these spices, good for you!!

Easy steps you can take right now

Get very friendly with someone from Asia or the West Indies. My friend is married to an Indian man so she gets to enjoy dishes made with these spices regularly.

Of course, it might be quicker to simply order some turmeric and/or curcumin online (or get it at your local health food store).

Move to London and get Indian takeout frequently.

Or, it's probably faster to buy an Indian food cookbook and make the delicious dishes yourself. My mouth is watering just writing about Indian food!

Ginger

Ginger has been used for so many centuries and for so many different ailments that I could devote a whole book just to this spice.

As I stated above, you can get turmeric combined with ginger if you have joint issues. It is a fabulous anti- inflammatory and anti- nausea agent.

Ginger is very pungent. If you don't cook with it, it can be challenging incorporating it into your diet.

Ginger can be made into a refreshing iced tea which is how I consume it. Get a piece of ginger root, peel it, slice a few pieces, throw in a cinnamon stick and boil for 5-10 minutes. Throw the water into a container and refrigerate. If you must add sweetener use Stevia or Luo Han.

Do not use any sugar - or even chemical sweeteners and sugar substitutes such as Sweet & Low or Splenda! Many studies are now showing that these artificial sweeteners may actually spike sugar as well as increase cravings for carbs![4] Both of these effects are kryptonite to people with diabetes. I personally can't see sabotaging all the beneficial actions for a yellow packet of poison.

Gotta say it again: Check with the doc if you choose to take ginger while on meds.

Make a plan to get a piece of ginger root, or get up and go do it now. Follow the instructions above to make iced tea.

Incorporate fresh ginger into your cooking by grating it into a nice veggie soup.

Berberine

Huh? Never heard of it? Neither had I until recently.

I was reading a very compelling "free" diabetes article - which of course turned out to be an upsell for certain products.

Again, let me state that I am not in any way affiliated nor am I compensated for any recommendations in this book.

The article mentioned some scientific terms I had never heard before. I realized that I could research the names and discovered some of the more common ones, such as turmeric.

However, there was one I had never heard of which turned out to be a supplement from the Barberry root.

Like cinnamon and turmeric, berberine (pronounced ber-ber-reen) has been used and touted for centuries as an important traditional medicine.

Berberine, as well as many traditional medicines, has been researched and validated by scientific communities. Researchers have discovered that berberine has the ability to naturally promote healthy blood sugar and metabolism.[5]

Healthy cholesterol levels as well as blood lipids are also among berberine's benefits. I always read reviews before deciding to try

---

[4] http://www.webmd.com/diet/news/20140917/artificial-sweeteners-blood-sugar#1

[5] http://articles.mercola.com/sites/articles/archive/2015/06/22/berberine-benefits.aspx

something, and as I read the reviews I was very impressed.

The people who wrote them very clearly stated that they had modified their eating AND exercised. I read that all their numbers were greatly improved and some reported the alleviation of diabetic neuropathy in their feet.

When I saw that this was a product in the Andrew Lessman lineup, I decided to give it a try. It was worth the research. I just ordered my second bottle.

Don't discount Berberine just because you've never heard of it. Remember Penicillin? The Wright brothers? Henry Ford? You get the picture. Do your homework and check with your doc.

Easy steps you can take right now

Google berberine and read up on it. If you feel encouraged by what you read, go to *www.procapslab.com* and order a bottle.

Make sure to follow the dosage on the bottle.

Moringa

Moringa Oleifera is also commonly known as moringa. Another plant most of us have never heard of. If you visit your local farmer's market, however, you likely will see someone selling it in pill and powder form.

Moringa is a fast-growing tree native to South Asia and now found throughout the tropics. Its leaves have been used as part of traditional medicine for centuries, and the Ayurvedic system of medicine associates it with the cure or prevention of more than 300 diseases.

Moringa is a super food whose leaves are loaded with vitamins, minerals, essential amino acids, and more. One hundred grams of dry moringa leaf contains:

- 9 times the protein of yogurt,
- 10 times the vitamin A of carrots,
- 15 times the potassium of bananas,

- 17 times the calcium of milk,

- 12 times the vitamin C of oranges,

- 25 times the iron of spinach... and many more health benefits.

Keep in mind that carrots, bananas, oranges, and other high sugar fruits and vegetables must be eaten in moderation if at all, especially when you are trying to control your sugar naturally.

While in Colombia several people had mentioned Moringa to me. My father-in-law eats Moringa seed for his diabetes.

He gave me one in the evening and within an hour my dinner was returning from both ends. Next time I google first and pop (or not) a seed after. I found out that the seed is super potent and should be eaten with extreme caution - if at all.

I recommend you try the pill form, as the powder form is a bit hard to take. The powder tastes a bit like a freshly mowed lawn thrown into a blender. You can mix it with a veggie smoothie or put it in a vegetable soup.

The benefits far outweigh the taste challenges. I got the powder at my local farmer's market. I was given a moringa plant and I harvest the leaves to blend with a vegan protein powder. I also use the powder form in a tea which makes it more palatable.

You know what I'm going to say now right? Check with the doc if you're also taking meds.

Easy steps you can take right now

Google moringa and read up on it. Then, if you want, order some on Amazon in pill form or tea form. Do your due diligence as to the product you order. It should be non-GMO, organic, etc...

Visit your local farmers market or health food store to buy moringa.

Alpha Lipoic Acid

People with diabetes or metabolic syndrome tend to do much better when taking lipoic acid, as it enhances insulin sensitivity.

There have been numerous studies on this powerful antioxidant as it relates to diabetes and other conditions as well.[6] People with tingling, pain, and numbness in their feet and legs have reported complete relief after only two weeks of taking this supplement.

It works by improving circulation. Lipoic acid has been found to reduce symptoms of lupus, rheumatoid arthritis, and other autoimmune diseases.

In a limited number of clinical studies, antioxidant drugs including alpha lipoic acid and vitamin E were found to reduce the symptoms associated with diabetic neuropathy.

As I write this, I have been taking alpha lipoic acid supplements for one week - and I am thrilled to tell you that I am already experiencing dramatic relief of pain in my feet and legs. Because my condition (Type 2) was long-standing and advanced, I had been experiencing symptoms for years and sometimes still do even though my sugar and A1C are way down.

I have every expectation that I will experience complete relief, since I have only been taking it for about a week and my foot and leg pain is almost 100% gone.

Now check this out: In Germany, doctors are *legally required to tell their diabetic patients about this supplement!*

Think about it. What are the moral ramifications of *not* telling patients that they can experience relief from such a debilitating symptom of diabetes with a natural product rather than a habit- forming narcotic? And yet we've all seen the commercials that warn about side effects ranging from mild nausea to becoming a werewolf during a full moon.

As with any supplement, check with your doctor first.

---

[6] http://www.webmd.com/diet/supplement-guide-alpha-lipoic-acid#1

Easy steps you can take right now

Remove all silver bullets from the house.

Once that's done, go to Andrew's website and order some Alpha Lipoic Acid.

Important side note: These supplements don't work while in the bottle. You actually have to take them.

Foot Cream

There are many creams on the market that promise to relieve tingling, burning, and pain in feet and legs. I have only tried one. It's called MagniLife Pain Relieving Foot Cream.

I love this stuff. It has provided me with incredible relief, especially at night. Combined with the Alpha Lipoic Acid, it has almost entirely alleviated all my symptoms in just a few days.

It's homeopathic and has even helped my husband who has suffered from Restless Leg Syndrome (RLS) for years. You just rub it on morning and night. It's moisturizing, non-greasy, and smells good too.

You can buy it at the drugstore (I got mine at CVS) for about $20. (If you get CVS rewards, as I do, you can buy it even cheaper with your coupon or discount.) There is also a buy 2 get one free on their website, www. magnilife.com.

If you are suffering from foot and leg pain, it's certainly worth a try at that price. For me, it wins hands down over any narcotic, habit forming pain relief drug.

Easy steps you can take right now

Get the cream! Do you enjoy tingling, numbness, or burning, in your feet and toes?

Acupressure

Acupressure is a type of massage in which finger pressure is applied on specific bodily sites. Acupressure is a therapy used to promote healing.

If you remember my experience in the airport in Panama, you might be very hesitant to try this. That's understandable.

However, if you are anything like me - meaning you want to heal your pancreas and stimulate them to produce insulin on their own (type 1), or help your cells absorb the sugar in your blood (type 2)—this is really a modality worth considering.

Acupressure is another modality based on the ancient Chinese practice of acupuncture without the needles.

The good news is diabetes can be controlled to a large extent if not totally reversed.

Tapping (see above) is a variation of both these techniques. I'm not including diagrams with the acupressure points as I strongly feel that you should consult a licensed practitioner to help you.

After a few visits, you can determine for yourself if acupressure is beneficial and you may practice it on your own.

My husband taught me the acupressure point for heartburn and nausea. It works every single time. He used to live on Tums... now he just applies pressure to that point for one minute and he gets instant relief.

I love that it is drug free and that, when done correctly, it can produce amazing results.

Acupressure may really make your doctor scoff. But I don't worry about that. After all, it's not his or her health on the line here. It's yours (and mine).

Just remember to tread carefully with acupressure if you are still taking meds. (Remember my airport experience?)

CBD Hemp Oil

CBD hemp oil may be the most controversial of all the supplements to consider. I have a good feeling about this one, and I have tried it for a short time... but I honestly can't say I've got much experience with it.

Read on and see if it's something you'd like to check out yourself.

Cannabidiol or CBD hemp oil is a natural botanical extract of the common hemp plant. CBD hemp oil is made from high levels of CBD, however it contains low-THC hemp.

THC is the compound in medical marijuana that is psychoactive. In other words, medical marijuana contains larger quantities of THC, while CBD oil contains very low amounts of THC but has great medicinal properties.

I took CBD oil from a dropper for a week or so and I can assure you that there are *no* psychoactive effects for me.

Dr. Sanjay Gupta (CNN Medical Correspondent) has done many specials on the positive effects of CBD oil, as has CBS' news show "60 Minutes." Look them up!

The medical community has made huge strides with scientific evidence touting the many healthful properties and health benefits of CBD oil.

The Stanley brothers in Colorado were highlighted on "60 Minutes" for the phenomenally beneficial effects of CBD oil in children with epilepsy and seizures. There are also significant studies being done with this treatment for cancer, Alzheimer's, and many other diseases - including, yes, diabetes.

The way CBD works is that it interacts with the body through the endocannabinoid system. In the late 1980s it was discovered that this system regulates the body's homeostasis (the fancy word for physiological balance).

This has an impact on functions such as immune response, pain, sleep, mood (anxiety and depression), appetite, and even hormone regulation. The endocannabinoid system regulates our bodies responses and restores balance.

If you would like to do your own investigation, you can google the Stanley

Brothers, or go to their Charlotte's Web site at **www.cwhemp.com**. The customer service is excellent and you can chat with a representative.

(By the way, shipping CBD hemp oil is *legal in all 50 states* so you don't have to worry about the FBI confiscating your cow mailbox!)

Now, CBD hemp oil is a bit pricey - and that, along with the fact that I've been doing so well using the other supplements and recommendations in this book, is why I didn't stick with it for very long.

However, CBD hemp oil is not nearly as expensive as the medical bills associated with unchecked diabetes. It's also got a lot of other benefits, so I do think it's worth checking out.

MCT Oil

Another friend of mine, a personal trainer, takes MCT (medium chain triglycerides) oil. MCT oil is a form of saturated fatty acids that also has numerous health benefits. It seems to have many of the same properties at CBD hemp oil.

She puts a tablespoon of MCT oil in her morning coffee. She says it's odorless and tasteless, and makes you feel full. It's a lot less expensive than CBD oil.

I ordered a bottle because I was curious to see if MCT oil could replace the hemp oil at a fraction of the price.

I have started putting a tablespoon in my decaf coffee... and she's right - it is undetectable. No odor or taste. It also really does make me feel full. I am also putting it on my dog's food at night as it's beneficial for joint health.

Easy steps you can take right now

Research the heck out of this one, then decide if you want to get one of them.

Cholesterol and Statins

Hold on to your seat belts. The next topic may be a bumpy ride for some of you.

There is a class of cholesterol medications known as statins. These include: Lipitor, Simvastatin, lovastatin, and others.

I did extensive research on this classification of drugs. What I found was highly disturbing.

All of the information came from respected medical institutions and I encourage you to do your own investigation.

Are your statins helping you... or someone else?

In a nutshell, I read that Lipitor is the most profitable drug in history, having profited more than *$125 billion* from 1997 to 2011.[7]

Yet this statin has been shown to not only be largely ineffective in lowering cholesterol.[8] It actually raises blood sugar![9]

There have now been over 64,000 reported cases of statins causing adult onset (type 2) diabetes. Those were *only* the cases that have been documented. The report went on to say that the financial rewards for medical professionals were so attractive that there is no way to stop these often-dangerous drugs from being prescribed.

Another reported side effect is the formation of cataracts. My husband has been on statins for years in spite of my constant nagging and warnings.

He just had a massive cataract removed from his eye and he is not in an age group often associated with this type of condition. He now needs a cataract removed from the other eye!

Did I need any more proof? I did not.

---

[7] http://www.crainsnewyork.com/article/20111228/HEALTH_CARE/111229902/lipitor-becomes-worlds-top-selling-drug

[8] https://www.nytimes.com/2016/04/04/health/dashing-hopes-study-shows-cholesterol-drug-has-no-benefits.html

[9] https://www.peoplespharmacy.com/2016/01/04/atorvastatin-lowers-cholesterol-but-raises-blood-sugar/

The medical community must be starting to take notice of the side effects because the last time I went to get a refill for my husband, the pharmacist flagged me down before I could walk away to ask me how long he had been on the medication AND if he had any muscle pain or other adverse side effects.

When I got home I noticed a warning in big red letters on the bag that contained the prescription about the muscle pain!!!

What to do if you have high cholesterol and diabetes?

I'm so glad you asked!

First and foremost...EXERCISE!! Yeah, I went there again. Get up and move as I've described earlier.

The good news is that once your blood sugar drops, more than likely so will your cholesterol.

Just a little aside here, I urge you to go to *www.mercola.com* and read what Dr. Mercola says about cholesterol. Many doctors now believe that cholesterol and heart disease have very little to do with each other.

Take care of yourself... but be careful who you trust.

Don't let the medical community tell you that you need dangerous and highly controversial drugs because your numbers are slightly over 200.

The medical profession has no incentive to send you to a qualified nutritionist or to suggest you try any other holistic healing modality.

Having said that, I will tell you that my cholesterol was close to 300... so I knew I needed to take something. I went to Andrew Lessman's website and ordered a natural cholesterol management product called Cholestacare with Fibermucil.

It is a combination of natural plant sterols and natural psyllium fiber. They come in convenient packets of 4 pills, which make them very easy to take with you when eating out or traveling.

The active ingredient has been so thoroughly researched for efficacy that it is the first natural ingredient to be recognized by the FDA for lowering bad cholesterol.

Diet and elimination

Along with this product - and exercise - I also incorporated more veggies and a bit less animal products into my diet.

I am not vegetarian or vegan. I didn't do anything drastic. I just cut down and certainly feel lighter.

Now, although it's not particularly pleasant to discuss... I have to share that my elimination system is also now working like never before.

Proper elimination is also crucial for overall health. Don't let your doctor tell you that none of this is connected. That's just pure bull!!

Diabetes affects *all* systems of your body. It's an inescapable fact.

My teeth

My last dental checkup was in May—before I knew about my sugar issue. For the last few years my hygienist kept having to inject my gums with antibiotics because there were very deep pockets and a lot of tartar build up on my teeth.

I would leave the office very disturbed and perplexed, as I have never smoked or used drugs.

Well, guess what? After only 5 months on my healthy new post-diabetes regimen, my teeth are in great shape!

The pockets in my gums have gone from 5-6 millimeters deep to only 3. No antibiotics for me anymore!

The hygienist told me that she had read about the link between diabetes and tooth decay but that she's never had a patient improve the condition of their gums and teeth the way I did with no meds.

Incidentally, my hygienist's father is a retired physician who refused to give her mother medication when she was diagnosed with diabetes. He took her to a holistic nutritionist - and she is now healthy and happy.

Another great benefit is that my dental visit co-pay was very minimal compared with the $40.00 per antibiotic I was paying before.

Lower blood sugar and healthy lifestyle saves you money.

That's a big bonus incentive for me!

My "unhealable" wound

Remember the wound on my shin that never closed? It looked like a scab that was only 50% healed. It never occurred to me that it was related to diabetes, talk about denial.

I thought I kept scratching it, or my dogs pawed me.

Nope.

Starve the body of sugar and watch the changes take place.

Easy steps you can take right now

Make the decision to eat less animal fat and more veggies.

Go directly to your computer and order the above recommended product.

Get off your behind and take a walk.

Decide to no longer be fooled by for-profit pharmaceutical corporations in spite of mountains of data to the contrary.

Now listen, I'm sincerely not on a mission to put drug companies out of business. But I am sincerely on a mission to show you your options and clear the path to health for you.

Chapter 10

Food

Let's make it very simple for everyone: No sugar!! That's it.

(OK, no, of course that's not it, but that's the most important rule about food.)

What about sugar substitutes?

Let me be perfectly clear on this topic.

Sugar means: white, brown, agave, honey, organic or not, to all the above, and all artificial sweeteners - except Stevia and Lo Han, a fruit from China.

Please don't think because you bought organic, local honey that you are safe. The same goes for brown sugar; this is sugar without the processing. Your body will react the same.

By now you know that *high fructose corn syrup—now also called "corn sugar"—is a health nightmare.*[10] It's all true. And you should read all labels

---

[10] http://drhyman.com/blog/2011/05/13/5-reasons-high-fructose-corn-syrup-will-kill-you/

because it is hidden in foods that you would never suspect would contain it—like bread, canned fruit, juices, and "energy" drinks, to name a few.

All of the above are more kryptonite to those of us with blood sugar challenges.

I promised you that you would stop craving all forms of sugar and I stick by that. However, you have to do your part and be committed to not eating it.

More and more drinks and food products are getting on the bandwagon and using Stevia, such as Crystal Light. I totally understand that drinking only water can get monotonous; we all want variety in our diet.

You can have it, but please just be aware of what's in your food and drinks.

Keep in mind that all sweeteners—artificial and natural—can spike your numbers as well as increase cravings for more sugar.

I know I said that earlier but I have to repeat myself to make sure you got it.

Sorry: No complex carbs for a while either.

Pasta, bread, rice, beans, corn, beets, potatoes, and sweet potatoes should all be eliminated from your diet while your body is healing.

These can be incorporated back in slowly after you regain your health. In the beginning though, these should all be avoided.

If you must eat carbs, keep it to no more than 20 grams per day. That's the equivalent to two slices of bread. This seems to be the magic number to stick to. When your carb intake is increased even a few grams beyond, your cravings will also increase which is what we want to avoid. I recommend you do follow a ketogenic diet (low carb, high in healthy fats).

Our task is difficult enough…don't make it any harder for yourself.

Fruit too??

Unfortunately, the same goes for most fruits. Bananas, melon, mangos, grapes, citrus fruits, and most berries all must be put aside for the time being.

At this point in my journey I am only eating half an apple about once per week. Sometimes I will put a little organic (no sugar) flax and chia seed butter on it that I buy at Trader Joes.

I can hear you cursing me. You may also be feeling overwhelmed because you think you're dying a culinary death.

Stop it!

There are loads of things you can still eat - and still maintain a healthy weight and blood sugar.

What kind of dairy is OK?

Here's the rule of thumb for dairy: The less fat in dairy, the more sugar they're putting into it.

I know. It goes against everything you've thought for years. But no fat and low-fat dairy is *not* the way to go. (But who cares, really? Skim milk might be the worst tasting thing on the planet anyway.)

My friend who puts the MCT oil in her coffee also puts in heavy cream. If you saw her body, you would believe me about full fat being okay.

No processed cheese, please. If you eat cheese, get the real deal and pair it with celery or make a nice tomato, cucumber, and feta salad with olive oil and white vinegar.

Feel free to eat full fat sour cream and cream cheese. Please make sure you buy these products in a pure, natural form. No preservatives or additives.

I would drop milk as it has sugar in it, but if you don't like almond, coconut or cashew milk, drink milk with no growth hormones or antibiotics. Of course, that's only in coffee or in a glass—because all your breakfast cereals, including sweetener-laden granolas and mueslis—have to be tossed or put way up on the shelf for now (literally). Again, milk may spike your numbers.

Remember, cereal includes oatmeal and grits, both of which spike sugar. And grits are made of corn, another no-no.

And when it comes to eggs, see below... but know that eggs are an egg-cellent form of protein despite the years of lies you've heard about them causing high cholesterol. They don't.

Nuts

Coconut anything is wonderful for your body - as long as it is not in a macaroon cookie. I use coconut for cooking, I put non-sweetened coconut milk in my soups, I even put the oil on my face at night as it is an excellent moisturizer and make up remover, even for mascara.

Same goes for macadamia nuts, walnuts, and almonds. These are all very healthy fats. When eaten in moderation they can be a superb snack alternative.

Olives are also excellent to add to salads or pop a few when you're feeling peckish.

What's for dinner?

Fish is the preferred protein for health benefits, but any protein is better by far than sugar/carbs. Eggs are also fabulous. Contrary to the myth about too much cholesterol, eggs are a fantastic source of protein unless you're a vegan.

Now, when it comes to dinner, I have learned to improvise and substitute in so many ways. All of them are simple and delicious.

For example, who doesn't love a big bowl of pasta? Buy a spaghetti squash, cut it in half, roast at 350 face down for 20 minutes, take a fork and shred the "meat" inside the halves. You will have a delicious alternative that you can mix with butter, olive oil, red sauce, or anything else you usually put on spaghetti.

Same goes for cauliflower. Boil until it's soft, whip it with milk or cream, add salt and pepper to make mashed "potatoes." A great alternative pizza crust is cauliflower, eggs, and parmesan cheese baked in the oven.

My Veggie Soup

My new best friend is now my veggie soup. I make a big batch on the weekend, and then I eat it all week long.

It's really easy. Just sauté an onion, a little garlic, a stalk or two of celery, and 1-2 chopped tomatoes (if you like) until soft, then put in 4-6 cups of veggie broth (I like it better than water and bouillon but you can use that if you want) with about 4-6 cups of any vegetable you like, cut up if you like. (I use zucchini, squash, spinach, brussels sprouts, string beans... but use whatever veggies you like best.) Bring it to quick boil then turn down the heat to simmer for 20-30 minutes or so. Voila!

It's filling, delicious, packed with nutrition... and there's no sugar!

If you like creamy soup, add some cream or coconut milk, get an immersion blender and blend until you have a delicious, creamy, healthy soup.

If you really can't stand the thought of cooking, go to any health food place and buy a few organic soups.

Lentil soup is great for people without blood sugar issues, but beware for now because it's a bit too high in carbs. Save it for down the road when your numbers are better. Stick to veggie soups and others with no pasta, rice, or beans for now.

Be prepared

This is so important I probably should have mentioned it first... preparation really is the key to eating right for diabetes.

You know the adage that you should never go grocery shopping hungry? Well, being hungry without appropriate food in the house usually leads to eating foods that are counterproductive to our mission.

Of course, you may be on the road, or too busy at times to be fully prepared. But do your best to have what you need in your fridge or in your car with you.

Eating on the road doesn't have to be disastrous. If you have to stop at a fast food joint, there are choices to replace burgers and fries. Get a salad with grilled chicken, a scoop of tuna, or no meat at all if you like. Choose a vinegar-based dressing with no sugar. Some places have veggie burgers on grain buns which is better than the alternative. Even better try a burger with a lettuce wrap instead of bread.

The reality is that most of us eat the same 5-10 foods from day to day. Just change what they are and make sure you prepare for the weeks and days ahead of you.

Oh, you're human? Me too.

If you do eat foods that are not recommended for keeping your blood sugar in check (holidays and special occasions) get back on track later that same day - no "I'll get back to it tomorrow" binging, please.

Most important: *Do not beat yourself up.* Throwing in self-loathing with your already challenging condition is unnecessary and counter-productive.

Let it go, and move on.

I just read a bombshell of an article!

In Dr. Mercola's daily newsletter which you can subscribe to for free, there is an article in the April 30, 2017 issue: *Courageous Doctor's Twitter Post Could Change Nutritional Guidelines Forever.*

In the University of Cape Town, South Africa a well-respected doctor, Dr. Tim Noakes was taken to court by the legal system to strip him of his medical license for promoting a low-carb diet.

I cannot suggest strongly enough that you read this article.

To summarize, Dr. Noakes feels that A low-carb, high-fat diet is crucial for preventing or reversing insulin resistance and type 2 diabetes. He also says that it is a huge mistake treating Type II with insulin. A position I am now coming across more and more from doctors.

Suffice to say that the science behind his theory was so compelling that he was vindicated in a South African court of law and before the medical community.

Easy steps you can take right now

Rid your pantry and fridge of all food that is counterproductive to your mission.

Make a list and/or go shopping for protein, veggies, and any other food that will help you to stay on the right path.

Cook a few things like the veggie soup, tuna salad, and a big bowl of salad stuff to eat for a few days.

Read the article.

Chapter 11

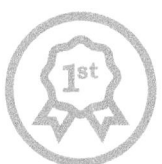

You First

So.

How do you feel?

I mean how do you *really* feel… about yourself?

There are lots of books about health. Unfortunately, not one of them can make you actually *care* about your health.

I have read hundreds of personal transformation books. Many of these books tell you that it's important to find your "why". In other words, what is your own true, deep down, personal and individual reason for wanting better health, money, a relationship, a particular job, etc.

This "why" question may seem irrelevant when you're talking about your physical well- being. But it isn't, believe me.

Diabetes is very complicated. It's not just about getting something you want. It's about very serious and unwanted physical consequences that you don't want. I certainly don't want any of them.

You Have To Be Your Own "Why"

I have a kid, a husband, family, friends, dogs, and all the other stuff that comes with having a life.

But I am doing this for me.

Not only because I want my daughter to have her mother here for as long as possible. I also want to be around for as long as I can.

And I don't want to just be "around" either. I want to *feel great* too, on as many days as I possibly can.

When I was first diagnosed, I identified myself as a "diabetic." But I stopped quickly - as soon as I realized that diabetes is something I have - it's NOT who I am.

It may sound funny, but the cells in your body have infinite intelligence within them. Despite what the medical community says, your cells know exactly *how to heal themselves.*

So please: Always keep in mind that what you *think* is just as important as what you *eat* and *do*. I have found that focusing on the healthy part of me, rather than the dis-ease part, has helped me tremendously.

I celebrate every disappearing symptom with an internal pat on my own back. I don't need praise and I am not obsessed with talking or thinking about it.

My greatest rewards are the improvements in my health.

I feel like a different person.

OK. So not every day is fantabulous, and I have had to make some adjustments. But I've learned to listen to my own body - and my own common sense. The best thing that my body did was *not* tolerating the medications. It forced me to take responsibility and find my own way.

My husband has a relative who has had diabetes for years. She talks of *nothing* else. When I try to discuss the steps I have taken and the improvements I've seen in only a few short months she says, "No one knows diabetes better than me."

She identifies so closely with diabetes that she has literally become the disease. She takes a specific kind of insulin, this medication may very well be killing people, according to the class action lawsuit commercials I have seen. She eats white flour, brown sugar, and just about everything on the do not eat list.

I can't convince her that there may be a better way. But that's OK. I want to "convince" by example.

That's why I wrote this book. I am doing it, and so can you.

My one and only intention is to provide information that may greatly improve your health, the quality of your life, and dare I say even prolong or save it.

If you feel overwhelmed, just start with what not to do.

Stop eating sugar. If that's all you do, BRAVO!

Then slowly incorporate any of the tips that seem doable and add as you see fit. Even I skip a day of exercising or taking all my supplements here and there.

And yes, I fall off the sugar wagon as well. I can tell you that I pay for it the next day with indigestion, constipation, fatigue, bad mood, and other lovely bodily conditions.

The good news is that I regain my feeling good status in a day or two. *The sugar rush is so not worth it.* You'll see what I mean when you cut out the sugar.

Approximately 9% of people in the U.S. have diabetes.

That's 29 *million* people in the United States alone.

And I'm supposed to believe that the medications are working wonderfully?

In a hilarious turn of events, my insurance company stopped covering 2 of the 3 meds prescribed for me. Without knowing it, they gave me yet another huge incentive to find a better way. A way in which I don't have to rely on anyone's "expertise" or ask anyone's permission to take control of my own body.

So right now, I am going to take my doggies for a long walk around a park with a lake.

Before I go, I'll close with a quote you need to read:

"Insanity is doing the same thing over and over, and expecting a different result."

~ Albert Einstein

Chapter 12

Resources and Info

Meditation, relaxation, stress, and sleep

www.youtube.com

Type in the search engine any of the above key words.

For meditation, search Deepak Chopra meditations, 15 minute meditations, or just meditation. Many options are available and you can choose the ones that appeal most to you.

Native American Flute music, chanting, or anything else that catches your eye.

Emotional Freedom Technique (EFT)

Google EFT for an explanation and the tapping points. Feel free to try any others that look interesting to you.

www.purposeprosperityhappiness.com (Helen McConnell)

www.bradyates.com

www.margaretmlynch.com (specializes in finances)

www.thetappingsolution.com

www.newfreedomcoaching.com (In Canada if you happen to live there, but you can do this remotely).

Exercise

Go to *www.youtube.com* and type in walking, yoga, aerobics, or any other exercise you are interested in into the search engine. Remember the "right" exercise is the one you'll do.

www.lesliesansone.com (Excellent for walking at home)

Buy a piece of exercise equipment like a treadmill, mini trampoline, bike, weights, etc., for home use. Hire a personal trainer if you can, they will keep you motivated and accountable.

Go to your local humane society website and volunteer to walk the dogs, or go ahead and rescue a dog. Walk the dog several times a day. You will not only get your exercise, you will find unconditional love with your new furbaby. (Yes, I'm a fanatic rescue dog person.)

Join a gym. Some are only $10.00 per month.

Start going for walks outside.

Any and all information you want to research regarding diabetes, nutrition, supplements, or any health related matter:

www.mercola.com

Type the subject you want to learn about into the search engine on the top right and read the related articles.

Dr. Mercola is a trusted, high reputable physician and a must read. I always reference him when I want the latest research and information. I also highly recommend his book *Fat for Fuel*.

You may find some of his ideas a bit radical. But then, penicillin and women voting were considered radical at one time.

Dr. Mercola does sell many products, some of which I have tried, but you don't have to buy anything to access his full library of fully-sourced health and nutrition articles.

Supplements

www.procapslabs.com

This is Andrew Lessman's company. You can also find his supplements on HSN (Home Shopping Network).

You will have to check the schedule for which supplements will be aired.

I usually go to Amazon because I have Amazon Prime which ships free for eligible products.

I get all of my supplements from Andrew Lessman with the exception of Moringa, as he doesn't carry it to the best of my knowledge.

Below are the supplements I buy from him:

- Cinammon

- Tumeric/Cumin

- Berberine

- Cholestacare with Fibermucil

- Alpha Lipoic Acid

Diabetic foot Nerve Pain

www.magnilife.com

You can buy this online or at your local drugstore. They usually have a buy two get one free deal. This company also carries products for arthritis and restless leg syndrome. They just added a product for migraines.

Acupressure

Google "licensed acupressure practitioners" in your area.

Interview them before making an appointment, and always ask them to send you their licensure.

Make sure they are experienced with diabetic patients, and check to see if they have any valid complaints about them. I always like to ask for actual client references anytime I hire anyone for anything.

CBD Oil

www.cwhemp.com

There are other sites, but this is the site of the Stanley Brothers. They have been on primetime shows and are the authority in pure hemp oil.

MCT Oil

www.sportsresearch.com

You don't have to be an athlete to enjoy the many benefits of this oil. I now put a tablespoon in my coffee or protein shake. It makes you feel full as well as being an extremely healthy fat.

Moringa

www.organicveda.com

You can also buy Moringa seeds online and grow your own tree.

Food

Stop eating sugar.

The American Diabetes Association guidelines are packed with carbs that we should not eat. I don't care what they say, they're wrong.

If you feel a nutritionist is right for you, find one that has up to date and extensive knowledge about appropriate food for people with diabetes.

Vegetables are great with the exception of carrots and beets.

Lay off the fruit for a while, when you do eat fruit choose low sugar ones.

Stay away from melons and bananas. Blackberries are okay in moderation.

If you eat apples, cut it in half and put some nut butter on it, or eat it with a piece of cheese.

Absolutely no fruit juice, especially store bought.

Drink water, tea, coffee (Stevia), make ginger tea with a cinnamon stick in it, or flavored seltzer water with no sugar.

Go to *www.mercola.com* and type in search bar "diabetic diet."

Organic dairy is best. Full fat sour cream and cream cheese, hard cheese or feta, almond or coconut milk with no added sugar.

Proteins include: eggs, poultry, meat, fish, and dairy.

If you're vegetarian or vegan you will have to modify your diet as pasta, rice, and beans are out.

Nut butters (no peanut butter) with no high fructose corn syrup or sugar. Macadamia and walnuts are best.

With a bit of effort you can find and eat good tasting and good for you foods.

Chapter 13

Recipes To Get You Started

Pasta

Cut a spaghetti squash in half, length wise

Cook on 400 for about 45 mins.

Shred the inside with a fork

Mix with butter, oil, red sauce, or anything you like on pasta that doesn't have sugar.

Mashed Potatoes

Boil a medium cauliflower in water until it is soft

Blend, ninja, or magic bullet

Add cream, garlic if you like it, salt and pepper to taste.

My Veggie Soup

Sauté in a little coconut oil:

Onions, garlic (fresh or from a jar), celery, zucchini, and squash.

Add a can of diced tomatoes (I like Rotel with habaneros to make it spicy) or chop fresh tomatoes.

Add vegetable or chicken bullion cubes (Low sodium if you have blood pressure issues) and any seasonings you like.

I like it spicy so I put in a teaspoon of hot sauce that my hubby makes.

Add two containers of vegetable or chicken broth (Also comes in low sodium)

I add a can of pure coconut milk which makes it a bit creamy and delicious

Add any other veggies you like. I put in:

Broccoli, green beans, cabbage and brussels sprouts.

As the soup begins to boil I add fresh spinach.

At this point I turn off the flame as the veggies stay fresh for a long time if you don't cook them to death.

I eat this soup all week. This has been a life saver on those days when I am very busy, tired, or just can't be bothered cooking.

Of course, you can always buy soup from a health food store but that gets expensive, and I make enough to last all week

Sauteed Onion and Egglant

If you're an eggplant lover (my husband would rather eat the cutting board) then you will love this simple, easy recipe.

Sautee an onion in oil, coconut oil, or even butter until brown.

Chop an eggplant into cubes and add to pan, cook until soft and brown

You can add mushrooms, broccoli, chicken, whatever else you want, or nothing at all.

In a Pinch

Keep some salad stuff in a container that you can throw in a bowl with oil and vinegar.

Buy salad in a bag but make sure it doesn't have sugary dressings or things like cranberries in it.

I buy zucchini pancakes made with vegetables from a company called Golden.

You can even get fake rice made from cauliflower already chopped in a bag. Saute with your favorite veggies for a stir fry.

Snacks

Celery sticks are excellent because they're crunchy. Add some no sugar nut butter or cream cheese, or a piece of hard cheese.

Macadamia nuts, and walnuts are all good sources of healthy fats, and filling. Please eat in moderation as they aren't calorie free foods.

Cucumbers with feta cheese, drizzle olive oil and a little salt.

Half an apple with a piece of cheese after your numbers are down.

Buy some dark cocoa powder and make your own hot chocolate with an alternative milk and Stevia.

Google veggie pizza with cauliflower crust, you will find easy, delicious recipes. Use the frozen cauliflower already "riced" for you.

As a matter of fact, there are thousands of easy recipes for those of us who need to avoid sugar and carbs.

And you thought you would have nothing to eat!!

Believe me your tastes will change. Give it a chance and put in the time and effort to find the foods you should and will eat.

FINAL THOUGHTS

Consistency is key.

I don't know how long it took to build Rome and I don't care.

I do know that the diabetes I have had for years according to the PA was well under control within 3 to 6 months.

If you think that's a long time, wait until you see how long your life seems with the effects of unchecked diabetes.

Wait until your health insurance decides you don't need the medications that were helping, if they were.

I don't know why you chose this book out of all the available information out there. I'm not going to get all metaphysical and say you chose this book for a reason.

But you did.

Maybe you chose this book because it's short and sweet (pun intended).

I'm not a researcher, scientist, or statistician, and I didn't want to overwhelm you with the mountain of information I sifted through.

I repeat, consistency is the key.

**"The key to getting
ahead is getting started."**

~ Mark Twain

ABOUT THE AUTHOR

Who I am not. I am not a diabetic. I am a person with a condition called diabetes. I am not helpless, I am not at the mercy of the mainstream medical community, or the pharmaceutical industry. I am not going to go quietly into the abyss of this condition.

Who I am. I am a person who makes choices every single day, hour by hour moment by moment concerning my behaviors. I am arming myself with all the latest, cutting edge information to live my life in a state of physical, emotional, and mental well-being. I am doing all I can.

I dedicate this book to all of us who choose the fish over the pasta in a restaurant, to taking a walk after dinner instead of sitting down to watch TV. To having the intestinal fortitude not to eat the sugary cereal in the house because it was a buy one get one free, you had a coupon, and your kids were having a few friends sleep over.

I am a "David" stacking the odds in my favor against a "Goliath." With each new day, I conquer the giant all over again.

Patrice Alevy